AKUAMMA

SEEDS

Learn how this African plant can increase brain stimulation, provide mood enhancement, and offer natural pain relief.

CHRISTOPHER KNOWLES

Printed in the United States of America

Statements made in this book regarding the herbal and natural products offered have not been evaluated by the food and drug administration as the FDA does not evaluate or test herbs. This information has not been evaluated by the US Food and Drug Administration, nor has it gone through the rigorous double-blind studies required before a particular product can be deemed truly beneficial or potentially dangerous and prescribed in the treatment of any condition or disease.

The information presented in this book is provided for informational purposes only, it is not meant to substitute for medical advice or diagnosis provided by your physician or other medical professional. Do not use this information to diagnose, treat or cure any illness or health condition. If

Table of Contents

Thank you for purchasing "Akuamma Seeds" we would like to offer you a free gift!! Visit http://www.earthlymist.com/products/ and enter AZSEEDS to receive 20% off your first THREE purchases of herbs, supplements and supplies.

History of African Medicine Versus Western Medicine

Medicine has been a part of society since the beginning of time. Each area, all over the world, differs in the methods in which they choose to treat certain symptoms and diseases. There are individuals who practice and treat patients with Western medicine; while there are others who prefer to use Eastern medicine. Whether, as an individual, you prefer the methods used in Western medicine or the methods in Eastern medicine, it is imperative to have adequate information regarding the benefits that both spectrums offer. Each type of medicine has a place in our society, and can provide benefits that fill in the gaps between the two. Let's take a look today at the Akuamma Seed, and the benefits that are associated with this herbal seed.

The World Health Organization (WHO) examined the percentage of individuals in third world countries that were still receiving traditional medicine over modern medicine. It was an overwhelming 80% of individuals in third world countries that were still receiving traditional medical care as their primary means of medical treatment. There are a few reasons as to why this percentage is so high. First, the individuals who live in these third world countries often are only able to receive medical care through traditional medicine for the simple reason that it is the only type of medicine offered. The second reason that those who live in these underdeveloped countries prefer this type of alternative medicine. These individuals prefer this alternative medicine because it offers benefits that modern medicine cannot provide. Individuals all over the world have their preferences when it comes to health care, and so it is largely based on personal preference. There are many individuals that prefer holistic approaches to medicine.

One of the major differences between Western medicine and African medicine is the basis in which diagnoses and treatment is carried out. In Western medicine we have created an environment in which patients who are feeling sick go to the doctor. The doctor then examines the patient as well as takes a comprehensive history that will explain the reason for the visit. The doctor then complies through lab testing, imaging, patient symptoms to determine the most likely diagnosis. After a diagnosis has been made then treatments are established. A majority of treatment plans include a variety of medications that have been approved by the FDA. The key to Western medicine is determining a cause of symptoms, and provide quantitative treatments that will provide results. African medicine focuses on the entire patient when determining the cause of illness, and then incorporating a treatment plan based on that information. In traditional African medicine the social, spiritual, physical, and mental well beings are considered when an illness presents. If symptoms arise and an individual is sick, in African medicine each of the areas are addressed and treated instead of only treating the physical symptoms of an individual. The treatment plan is based mainly on herbal medicines and a holistic approach to treatment. Akuamma Seed is one herbal approach that is being used in traditional African medicine. It is being used in a variety of ways to treat a variety of illnesses and symptoms. It has been used in African medicine for many years. Let's take a look further into the benefits of Akuamma Seed

What Is Akuammine/Akuamma Seed?

Picralima Nitida is a tree that is naturally found in the forests of Africa. Countries including: Ghana, Ivory Coast, Nigeria, and more have these trees that produce Akuamma Seeds (Iwu, 1993). Akuamma Seed also known as Picralima Nitida comes from the family Apocynaceae. The alkaloids that compose the Akuamma Seed include: Akuammidine, Akuammine, Akuammicine, Pseudoakuammigine, and Akuammigine. There are other components that make up the Akuamma Seed; however, these are the five alkaloids of interest that we will be discussing. It is an alkaloid with several components of interest. Each of the alkaloids play an important role in the functioning of the Akuamma Seeds. The main uses that have been documented include the treatment of: fever, hypertension, jaundice, and malaria. These are the recommended uses of this particular herbal seed. However, there has been several testimonials from individuals who have claimed that the Akumma Seed and Akuammine have analgesic effects and are useful in treating painful conditions. This is a separate debate and we will try to address the facts concerning Akuammine and the Akuamma Seed.

Akuamma Seeds are gathered from a tree that is native to Western Africa. These seeds are gathered and dried and then consumed in other parts of the world. Akuamma contains many alkaloid components and the major one that is of interest is the

Akuammine. Akuammine comprises the majority of these seeds. It is used in parts of the world as a pain medication. However, the uses that have been documented do not include analgesia. Therefore, the information must be further researched in order to determine the potential benefits and risks associated with this seed. Akuammine has been labeled as an opiate but functions by binding mostly kappa opioid receptors. It actually acts as an opiate antagonist to the mu opiate receptors. There are three types of opioid receptors that the human body possesses. Those receptors are mu, kappa, and delta. There are many different benefits and side effects that occur when any of these opioid receptors are bound. Kappa opioid receptors can actually have negative effects and create a sense of dysphoria, unlike an opiate that binds to mu receptors which produces other effects. Akuammine is considered to be a strong analgesic as compared to the other alkaloids. It however, is thought to act by activating the sympathetic nervous system which results in fight or flight like symptoms. Because it is an opiate, it does result in constipation. Opiate receptors are also present in the intestines and because these are non-selective components, they will bind receptors in all areas of the body in which there are opiate receptors. These alkaloids bind the opiate receptors in the gut and thus results in strong constipation, and can even result in paralysis of the intestines. Because it does in fact still bind any type of opioid receptor, it does offer pain relief and suppression of certain illnesses that may be present.

The next alkaloid Akuammidine also acts as an opiate, but tends to bind to all the opiate receptors. Those receptors include the mu, delta, and kappa receptors. The activity is very weak, and has a very little binding capacity. It has the highest binding capacity to kappa receptors which offer some benefits. The effects of this alkaloid include: muscle relaxant and treats high blood pressure. Because it is an opiate analgesic it does offer some analgesic effects. The traditional opiates that are prescribed in Western Medicine normally bind to the mu receptors with great affinity. The mu opiate receptors are those that provide pain relief as well as provide the euphoric effect that can have the potential to be abused. Akuammidine binds weakly to the mu receptors, so there is little of this type e of effect when taking Akuammidine. The Akuammidine alkaloid binds more tightly to the kappa receptors, and this results in some analgesic effects, but can also result in dysphoria. Each alkaloid is similar but has different variability in the effects and benefits that they offer.

The third alkaloid is Akuammicine. Akuammicine binds to the opiate receptors and is and is also sometimes used as an analgesic. It binds to kappa opiate receptors and thus does not provide the euphoria that is normally present with opiates. Because it actually binds to kappa receptors, there is a high chance that the alkaloid will result in dysphoria. Dysphoria is an unwanted side effect that can deter abuse potential, while also allowing for pain relief. There is still studies to be performed in order to identify if the binding capacity is partial or full. Studies have indicated that in certain animals the binding capacity is interpreted as full kappa agonist, while in others this alkaloid is only a partial agonist. Therefore, further testing is required before determination of its benefits and side effects.

Pseudoakuammigine also provides analgesic effects. As with all the other alkaloids we have discussed, there is significant variability in which they are able to bind the opioid receptors. Pseudoakuammigine is unique as compared to the other alkaloids. One unique benefit that Pseudoakuammigine offers in addition to binding to opiate receptors, is that is also provides anti-inflammatory benefits. there is definitely more room for additional studies to take place in order to better understand the effects of this particular alkaloid. Through current studies there have been promising results that indicate the usefulness and benefits associated with this particular alkaloid. There have been some minor studies that have concluded that this particular alkaloid can have effects on both components of the nervous system. The two components of the nervous system include the Parasympathetic and the Sympathetic. The parasympathetic nervous system is responsible for what is known as "rest and digest." When an individual is in the Parasympathetic mode, they will experience the following: increased gut motility, decreased respiration, decreased heart rate, decreased blood pressure, and decreased metabolism.

The Sympathetic portion of the nervous system is responsible for what is known as, "fight or flight" response. When an individual is in the Sympathetic mode they will experience symptoms such as: increased heart rate, increased blood pressure, hyperventilation, and diminished gut activity. There are many benefit associated with Pseudokuammigine. With all the benefits, there are also associated risks; therefore, it is imperative that further testing be completed in order to determine the full spectrum of risks versus benefits.

Akuammigine is the final alkaloid that we will discuss. Akuammigine, thru a variety of testing, has shown very minute promising results. It does not offer the same analgesic effects as seen with the other alkaloids that compose the Akuamma Seeds. One benefit that Akuammigine is beginning to show is its antagonistic effect on epinephrine. Epinephrine is a hormone that is released in the human body. Epinephrine is released from the adrenal gland and when it is released creates a "fight or flight" response. It basically jumpstarts and is responsible for the symptoms that are present with the Sympathetic nervous system is activated. Because it acts against these effects, Akuammigine actually can exude benefits on areas in the body that have those specific receptors. When Akuammigine binds these receptors that antagonize Epinephrine, the results mimic the Parasympathetic nervous system effects. Akuammigine binds receptors in the heart and in the blood vessels, so the benefits can be tremendous if the right scientific studies can prove its effectiveness. Now that we have established the components that actually comprise the Akuamma Seeds, we can realize how important each of these alkaloids play in treating pain, high brood pressure, diarrhea, malaria, and many other symptoms and diseases. There is great opportunity for further research to conclude the benefits associated with this therapy that has been used consistently in Eastern medicine.

These Akuamma Seeds are used as a form of medicine in Africa. These Akuamma Seeds are a part of the Picralima Nitida tree. The seeds are composed of several alkaloid compounds that offer a wide spectrum of benefits. This form of treatment has been used in traditional African medicine for decades. Those who have received this treatment in Africa, have observed first hand the benefits that these seeds have on a variety of diseases and symptoms. The Akuamma Seeds are also used to treat a variety of symptoms and diseases. A few that have been documented are: malaria, diarrhea, diabetes, and fever. It is also thought to offer anti-inflammatory benefits as well as analgesic benefits.

How is it obtained?

Akuamma Seeds come from a tree that is naturally found in West Africa. The seeds from this plant are then dried and used for medical purposes in West Africa. These Akuamma Seeds are used as a form of medicine in the treatment of many patients in West Africa. These Akuamma Seeds are obtained through crushing and drying the seeds. The seeds are then taken orally. It has been reported through testimonies that the Akaumma seeds can act as opioids, and therefore, can be beneficial in the treatment of severe pain. There is very little evidence, other than information received from patient experience to indicate that Akuamma Seeds have these analgesic effects. There has been no scientific data, or clinical trials that have indicated any validity to the use of Akuamma Seeds for the treatment of pain.

As we stated in the beginning Akuamma Seeds are comprised of alkaloids. The alkaloid that we are most interested in delving deeper into its understanding is the alkaloid Akuammine. It is the major component in the seeds and makes up over half of the entire seed structure. These seeds are gathered from the Picralima Nitida tree.

The seeds are then crushed and made into a powder and in African medicine is consumed. It can be placed in a capsule in order to swallow as a pill. In the United States, it is not for human consumption at this time. The reason is there have not been the clinical trials that are required in order to receive FDA approval. The tree offers a variety of benefits. For instance, the bark of the Picralima Nitida tree actually has anti-parasitic benefits. The pulp of the Picralima Nitida tree is thought to offer benefits to those who suffer from hyperglycemia. The entire Picralima Nitida tree offers herbal medical benefits for a variety of diseases. Now that we have established the medical benefits of Akuamma Seed, let's take a further look into the diseases that Akuamma Seeds show promising benefits in treating.

What Diseases Do Akuamma Seeds/Akuammine Treat?

Akuamma Seeds offer a variety of benefits in the treatment of many different diseases and symptoms. Akuamma Seeds have been linked to addressing the following diseases and symptoms: pain, anti-malaria, hyperglycemia, fever, diarrhea, high blood pressure and many others.

As we have discussed above, Akuamma Seeds are composed of a variety of alkaloids that bind to opiate receptors. Because the Akuamma Seeds bind to opiate receptors, these seeds provide analgesic benefits to those who are suffering from painful conditions. One of the major concerns in our country today is how to treat chronic pain. Chronic pain is an issue that is constantly being discussed in the medical literature and in clinical practice. There is so many alternative therapies that are being implemented to try to address this issue of chronic pain. Akuamma Seeds offer a natural, herbal treatment that can allow for pain relief. Akuamma Seeds are different than other opiates in that most of the alkaloids bind to kappa and delta opioid receptors versus the mu receptors that create "the high" that so many drug abusers seek. The Akuamma Seeds offer analgesic effects.

A journal article titled, "Pseudo-Akuammigine, an alkaloid from Picralima Nitida seeds, has anti-inflammatory and analgesic actions in rats" written by M. Duwiejua, E. Woode, and D.D. Obit. The journal article was published in 2002 in the Journal of Ethnopharmacology. The article reviews the benefits associated with Picralima Nitida seeds (Akuamma Seeds). The study examined the benefits of Akuamma Seeds in rats who were induced with paw edema. Rats were being tested, had an animal population. The testing was completed using rats. Those rates were then induced with specific physical signs that were then treated using Akuamma Seeds. The main factor in this testing using rats, was to determine the effects of Akuamma Seeds on paw swelling. The results of this study showed that, "Pseudo-akuammigine therefore exhibits anti-inflammatory and analgesic actions. The analgesic actions are mediated via interaction with opioid receptors" (Duwiejua, Woode, Obiri, 2002). Having an alternative herbal medicine that offers this extensive pain relief, provides hope to those individuals who suffer from chronic pain on a daily basis. There are a lot of individuals in our society today that do not want to put synthetic, toxic pharmaceuticals into their bodies because of the negative outcomes that are associated. When they determine that Akuamma Seeds have strong pain relieving properties it provides hope to those who have chronic pain.

Akuamma Seeds have also been shown to have anti-plasmodial effects. Malaria is still a disease that affects many countries. It is not a disease that has diminished over time. It is a disease that is still affecting the population. According to the World

13

Health Organization (WHO), "Malaria is a life-threatening disease caused by parasites that are transmitted to people through the bites of infected female Anopheles mosquitos" (WHO, 2016). Malaria affects those all over the world, but affect those who live in underdeveloped countries more often. It is still a disease that is very prevalent in Africa. The World Health Organization (WHO) continues to declare Africa as the continent that has the highest malaria diagnoses still to this day. Sub-Saharan Africa was home to 88% of those who were diagnosed with malaria. Sub-Saharan Africa was also had the highest mortality rates of those who contracted malaria. The mortality rate according to the World Health Organization was 90% in Sub-Saharan Africa (WHO, 2016). As you can see, malaria is a parasitic infection that is still reeking havoc on the population of those around the world. The important factor concerning malaria is that it is completely preventable. There are preventative measures that can prevent individuals from every having this disease. The reasons that individuals normally are infected with malaria include: being unaware that they are exposed to the disease, unprepared foreign travel, residents of third world countries in which many live outside, and finally unable to afford insect repellant or bed nets for protection from mosquitos. These are just a few of the reasons that individuals can potentially be exposed to malaria.

Malaria is a very smart infection. What I mean by that, is that it uses the human bodies own cells to replicate and develop further. In order to better understand malaria, we need to evaluate the life cycle of this disease. Malaria is a parasite that infects the cells of humans. It is transmitted via the Anopheles mosquito. The mosquito bites the human and transmits the parasite. The mosquito injects the sporozoites into the human and that initiates the life cycle of the parasite. The malaria parasite multiplies in the liver cells and the red blood cells. The replication cycle continues in the red blood cells, and daughter parasites continue the life cycle of the parasite by infecting other red blood cells. The parasite continues to grow and now the patient begins to exhibit symptoms. The replicated parasite in the human blood is then ready for the mosquito to take that blood through another bite and continue the transmission of this disease. Once the mosquito bites an infected human, the gametocyte grows and replicates in the mosquito producing sporozoites in the salivary glands of the mosquito. As the mosquito bites another human, the life cycle of the parasite begins again (CDC, 2016). It is a devastating disease that can be prevented with the appropriate prophylactic care. The symptoms that are associated with malaria include the following: fever, chills, sweats, headache, nausea and vomiting, body aches, malaise, enlarged spleen, jaundice, and enlarged liver (CDC, 2015). These symptoms can result in secondary negative outcomes that can result in hospitalization and even death in some instances. Therefore, it is imperative that there be safe treatment options that will allow for the effective eradication of this parasitic infection. Akuamma Seeds offers an alternative to modern Western medicine. Akuamma Seeds are being tested in animal studies and are proving to be a real contender in the treatment of malaria.

Akuamma Seeds have been tested in animals, and the results are showing promising results when treating malaria. In the Journal of Ethnopharmacology, an article titled, "Evaluation of antiplasmodial activity of ethanol seed extract of Picralima Nitida" written Jude Okokon, B.S. Antia, A.C. Igboasoiyi, E.E. Easier, and H.O.C. Mbagwu. The study was also completed in animals, and the outcomes that were trying to be reached included determining if Akuamma Seeds were an alternative treatment for malaria. The study was conducted in mice. The mice that were participating in the study were infected with Plasmodium berghei berghei. Plasmodium berghei berghei is a specific strain of malaria. The Akuamma Seeds were given within a recommended dosage range between 35 and 115 mg/kg/day based on the weight of the mice. After the infected mice were treated with the recommended dosage of Akuamma Seeds, it was noticed that there was significant schizonticidal activity during the early infection stage as well as in established infection (Okokon, et. al, 2007). The study was conducted in vitro in mice. The results were very promising. The only issue with the results is that they were not better than the current anti-malarial drugs that are currently used in Western medicine. The standard of care is treatment with therapeutic pharmaceutical agents such as Chloroquine. However, for those individuals who have extenuating circumstances this can be a very beneficial treatment. Extenuating circumstances can include but are not limited to: living in a third world country in which modern Western medicine is not available, being unable to afford the cost of these medications, or choosing to use herbal methods to treat malaria and prevent exposure to toxic medications that can result in devastating side effects. Some individual decide that alternative medicine, or herbal medicine is able to provide benefits that are natural and do not exhibit the toxic side effects that the modern medicine standard of treatments have on our population. These effects prove that there is important medicinal uses for the Akuamma Seeds. Not only are the Akuamma Seeds proving to be important in treating parasitic infections, but there is also promise in these seeds providing an alternative treatment method for Diabetes Mellitus.

Diabetes Mellitus is a disease that has become quite prevalent over the past several years. Type II Diabetes Mellitus is very common today, especially in the United States. With the increase in the obese population across the United States, Type II Diabetes Mellitus continues to rise uncontrollably. Type II Diabetes Mellitus results in insulin resistance. It is completely preventable, and reversible if the individual looses the appropriate amount of weight. Type II Diabetes Mellitus occurs because the pancreas is consistently overproducing insulin, and then over time, the cells that produce insulin become resistant and no longer respond to the increase in blood glucose levels.

Without the proper production of insulin, the sugar levels begin to increase in the blood. The increase in sugar in the blood can result in detrimental and devastating effects. Kidney failure, peripheral neuropathy, diabetic coma, unable to heal from infections or wounds are just a few of the devastating effects that Diabetes can have on the human body. Treatment of this condition is absolutely necessary. For those who suffer from Type II Diabetes Mellitus, the first and foremost recommendation is lifestyle changes. It is imperative that lifestyle changes be implemented so that this disease can be reversed. In the meantime, medical treatment is necessary to prevent this disease from progressing. Modern Western medicine is very effective in treating Diabetes Mellitus; however, there are significant side effects that can be experienced. Therefore, an alternative that offers the same benefits without all the side effects is a very important medical breakthrough that must be addressed. Akuamma Seeds are showing very promising results as an alternative therapy for treating Type II Diabetes Mellitus.

An article published in the Phytochemistry Letters titled, "Glucose uptake stimulatory effect of akuammicine from Picralima nitida (Apocynaceae)" by Hafsat Shittu, Alexander Gray, Brian Furman, and Louise Young. The study that was conducted showed that the alkaloid Akuammicine stimulated the uptake of glucose in mature adipocytes (Shittu, et. al, 2010). Adipocytes are fat cells. Because the sugar was taken up by cells instead of being absorbed in the blood, the result in a regulated and maintained blood sugar level. These seeds have been a form of treatment for many years in Africa. Nigeria was one of the countries in Africa that seemed to implement the uses of the Akuamma Seeds in order to provide the benefits of reducing blood glucose levels to those who suffered from Diabetes. These are huge break through results that offer great potential to those who wish to use alternative treatment methods to treat their Diabetes. Diabetes is a disease that affects millions. It is a disease that can result in devastating outcomes including death. Therefore, having an herbal medicine that will be available to those who cannot afford it is very beneficial especially to those in third world countries.

Akuamma Seeds have shown very promising results when treating malaria, Diabetes Mellitus Type II, and pain. These are just a few of the diseases and symptoms in which there have been scientific evidence that proves these benefits. The benefits have been proven through animal studies. More importantly, these treatment methods have been routinely used in African traditional medicine. Alternative therapies have the opportunity to offer benefits that modern Western medicine cannot. Those in Africa have been able to reap the benefits of this herbal medicine, and in the Western world we are just now observing the benefits that they have known for years.

Other Medical Benefits of Akuamma Seeds

As we have discussed the entire Picralima tree offers a variety of medicinal benefits. According to the book titled *Handbook of African Medicinal Plants,* "In Central Africa, it is used for the treatment of primary hypertension, malaria, and jaundice. The crushed seeds are eaten for stomachache and pneumonia. Extracts of the stem bark and seeds are administered for general diseases and as a vermifuge" (Iwu, 1993). The Akuamma Seeds are also thought to be an herbal treatment for those who suffer from sleep disorders.

There is not much research to suggest the specific mechanism of action in which how this herbal medication works; but there are links to these specific benefits. More evidence is needed in order to prove that the Akuamma Seeds provide these benefits. However, the results are being produced in Africa, and so that information can be translated into research that is being conducted here in the United States. Over time, the benefits of Akuamma Seeds will be proven through research.

What is the legal status of Akuamma Seeds/Akuammine?

The legal status is something that has been controversial for years. There have been articles written trying to determine the legal status of Akuamma Seeds. The information that has been identified is two-fold. The first determination of this herbal medicine's legal status is when evaluating it in the context of where it is most used: Africa. In Africa, it is completely legal. The Akuamma Seeds, as we have stated above, is used in traditional African medicine to treat a variety of symptoms and diseases. It has been used for hundreds of years and has proven to be an effective means of alternative therapy.

Trying to determine the legal status of this herbal medicine in the United States was a little more difficult. What I have found, is there are multiple websites that offer to sell these Akuamma Seeds. However, if you read the fine print, located at the bottom of most of them; you will find there is a disclaimer that states not for human consumption. Even though there has been significant research conducted on the benefits that this alternative therapy offers, it still has not been FDA approved. In order to be FDA approved, there has to be double-blinded, randomized, controlled trials that create a non-bias study. These clinical trials then progress from phase I to phase IV, in which participants are followed over a significant period of time.

Because the appropriate protocol has not occurred for the Akuamma Seeds, it is not FDA approved.

The legal status is not really known. There are websites that sell these seeds; however, there has been little legislation that has either deemed these alkaloids illegal.

Dosing and Preparation

Because this is an herbal medicine and not a traditional medicine that is prescribed by a physician and obtained from a pharmacy, there is little information that provides reliable and valid dosages for this particular herbal remedy. There is specific information that provides dosages that have been thought to be effective. However, because they are not of a reliable source, it is not reputable enough to place in this documentation.

It is imperative that if you are wanting to look further into the benefits and treatment with Akuamma Seeds, to speak with a Naturalistic or Holistic physician. These individuals who have had extensive training in the areas of natural and holistic medicine can provide the recommended dosages for these herbal remedies. In some instances, there may not be enough evidence to treat a disease or symptom with this specific herbal remedy.

Through the literature, the majority of those in Africa who received this treatment received it orally by crushing the seeds into powder and then consuming them. This method does not specifically give the recommended dosages; however, it seems to offer many benefits so more standardized clinical trials are needed to establish a safe and effective dosage for the population.

Future Research

The Picralima Nitida tree has been a part of history for years. It has offered many medicinal benefits from its bark to its seed. The particular component of the Picralima Nitida that we have been interested in today was the Akuamma Seed. After reviewing the literature and the information from herbal medicine journals and textbooks, we have learned that there is definitely a reason to continue to research the Akuamma Seed.

These seeds offer so many benefits and have been a part of traditional African medicine for years. Africa is where this Picralima Nitida tree is native to. In Africa, Akuamma Seeds are used as a form of treatment for many different diseases and symptoms. We have seen through the research above, that Akuamma Seeds offer medicinal benefits in treatment of pain, malaria, fever, high blood pressure, and Diabetes Mellitus Type II. These are just a few of the diseases and symptoms that Akuamma Seeds have been shown to exhibit positive outcomes.

Akuamma Seeds are the seeds from the Picralima Nitida tree. These seeds are composed of several alkaloids that bind to the opiate receptors in the body. There have been studies conducted that prove the beneficial effects of Akuamma Seeds in treating pain because of its ability to bind to the opiate receptors.

The five alkaloids that compose the Akuamma Seeds each offer a variety of properties that is unique. Some of these alkaloids bind to the mu opiate receptors, while other bind to the kappa or delta opioid receptors. Pseudoakuammigine not only was responsible for providing pain relief via the binding to the opioid receptors, but also proved to offer anti-inflammatory benefits. These anti-inflammatory benefits were shown through animal studies. As we discussed, there was a clinical trial that looked at rats and in those rat's paw edema was introduced. After the administration of Pseudoakuammigine the swelling in the rat's paw was reduced, thus proving its ability to offer anti-inflammatory capabilities. Akuammicine, as we discussed, not only has the pain relieving properties, because of its capability to bind to the opioid receptors; but also, its ability to result in increased uptake of glucose in the adipocytes has proven effective in treating Diabetes Mellitus Type II. Each of these alkaloids offer analgesic effects, while also providing their own unique benefits. These diseases are present in our society. They should not have such an effect on our population.

The other parts of the Picralima Nitida tree showed promising results for treating a variety of illnesses and symptoms as well. While we did not go into depth, covering the benefits, I think it is imperative to take notice of just how beneficial this tree is to the traditional African medicine. The tree bark can be placed in boiling water, and the benefits are tremendous against parasitic and protozoan infections. One major parasitic infection is Chagas disease. Chagas disease affects thousands on a yearly basis. The mortality rate of this disease is also in the thousands on a yearly basis. Therefore, if there is a natural herbal medicine that can allow for prevention and treatment of this disease, then there is great hope for those who are unable to receive modern Western treatment. The pulp portion of the Picralima Nitida tree has also been used in traditional African medicine. It has been used to treat high blood sugars as well. These are benefits that need to be used not only in traditional African medicine, but also in the Western medical world. These Akuamma Seeds offer a wide spectrum of benefits, and as such further research is warranted to prove those benefits so that the components of these Akuamma Seeds can become FDA approved and used in the United States as a standard of care treatment.

Because the Akuamma Seeds are used in traditional African medicine, there are decades of real life implementation that have proven the benefits of this seed. However, in the United States there has been little literature that have proven the effectiveness. The clinical trials that have been conducted have been in animals and not in humans. Therefore, there is a need for significant research before any further action can be taken with these Akuamma Seeds.

When it is safe for these clinical trials to move from animal trials into human trials, the process of FDA approval can begin. When these clinical trials begin the approval process, there will be 4 phases that have to be completed successfully in order to become approved. After it has completed phase IV, then there will be much more information that will address the risks versus the benefits of the Akuamma Seeds. Right now, we only know what is being told to us from the traditional African medicine. We are unable to quantitatively gather the research to prove beyond a shadow of a doubt that these seeds will provide these benefits for this particular population. Therefore, a disclaimer must be placed stating that results will vary. In the United States, most websites that are trying to sell these seeds state that they are not for human consumption. There is no regulation on these seeds, so it is imperative that proper research be done before consuming these seeds. Please speak to an expert in traditional African medicine, or a physician in Naturalistic or Holistic medicine that may be able to provide more information regarding the safety of these Akuamma Seeds long term. There are risks to every drug, no matter if it is herbal or prescription. Therefore, make sure that you do your due diligence to determine the benefits versus risks associated with the Akuamma Seeds.

From the limited research that has been conducted, the benefits are very present. These Akuamma Seeds will be able to provide promising results for the future of medicine. Traditional

African medicine has been reaping the benefits of these alternative medicine therapies. Now that we have learned from their research, we can truly say that Western medicine can take a page from the alternative medicine therapies, because they offer significant benefits.

Conclusion

As we look to the future of medicine, I believe there is going to be a closure in the gap between Eastern medicine and Western medicine. There have been herbal remedies that many have devoted their lives to proving their benefits. There have been countless clinical trials proving the effectiveness of Western medication as a standard of care in many diseases. Therefore, the combination of the two spectrums of medicine, can provide the patient with the best outcome. With every drug there are side effects, so incorporating natural and herbal medicines can help alleviate and be offered as an alternative to those pharmaceuticals that result in serious negative outcomes. With the continued research on Akuamma Seeds, we can look to determine the long term benefits that this herbal medicine has to offer. The future of medicine looks bright.

Sources were gathered from the following websites:

http://www.naturalether.com/?product=akuamma-seeds-picralima-nitida

http://www.allaboutheaven.org/suppression/66/115/picralima-nitida

http://www.ancient-origins.net/history-ancient-traditions/traditional-african-medicine-and-its-role-healing-modern-world-004522

http://www.sciencedirect.com/science/article/pii/S037887410200582

http://www.who.int/mediacentre/factsheets/fs094/en/

http://www.sciencedirect.com/science/article/pii/S037887410600623

https://www.cdc.gov/malaria/about/biology/

http://www.cdc.gov/malaria/about/disease.html

http://www.sciencedirect.com/science/article/pii/S18743900
09001104

https://books.google.com/books?id=LMfMBQAAQBAJ&pg=
PA278&lpg=PA278&dq=akuamma+seeds+in+treatment+of
+malaria&source=bl&ots=Vx2bF472d8&sig=BE0EteDusuY
84A9W4tlx3greF-
4&hl=en&sa=X&ved=0ahUKEwi36sLC98HPAhUEGB4KHX
NDAyoQ6AEILDAH#v=onepage&q=akuamma%20seeds%
20in%20treatment%20of%20malaria&f=false